THAT'S THE JOB FOR ME!

I'M GOING TO BE A DOCTOR!

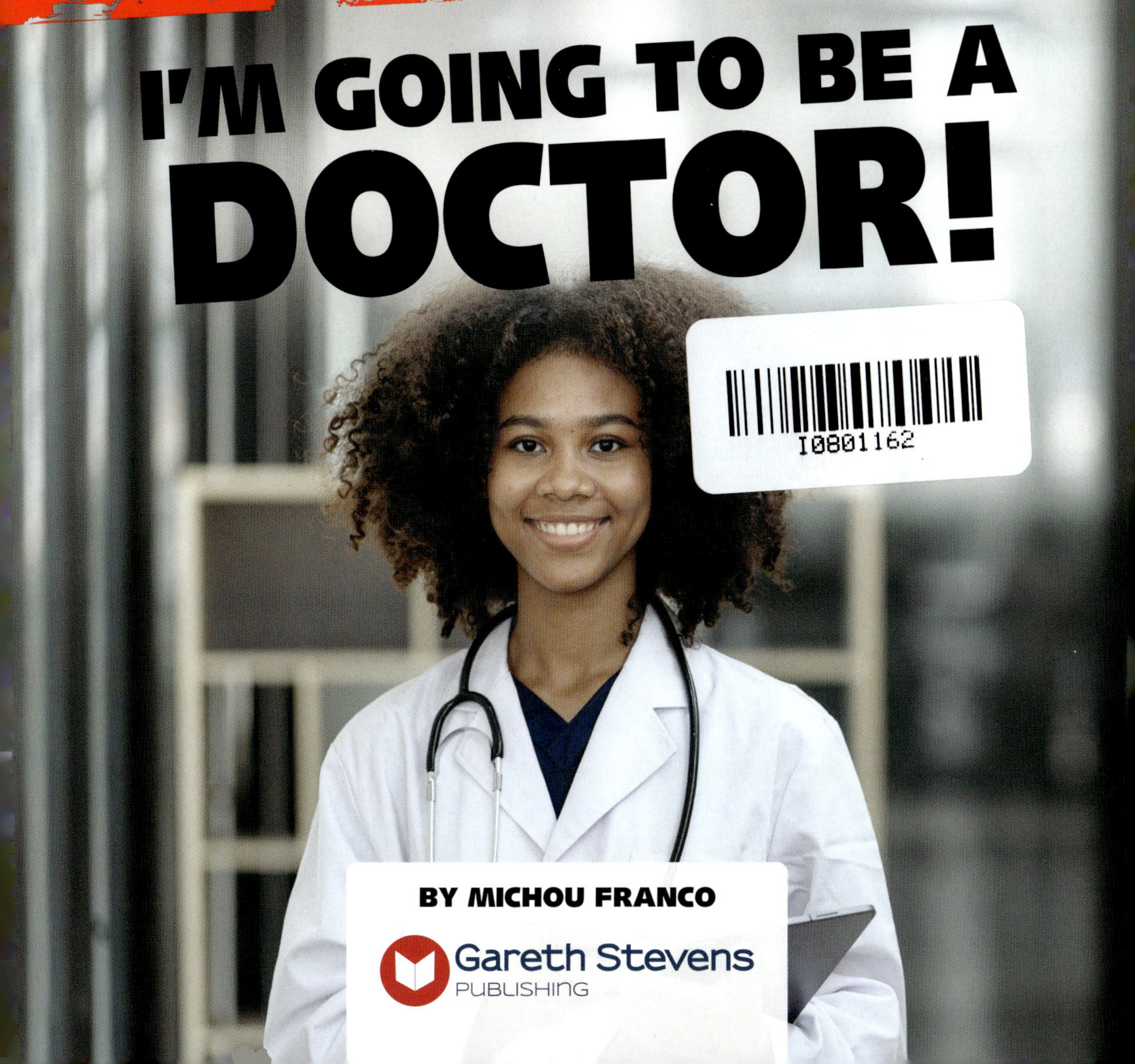

BY MICHOU FRANCO

Gareth Stevens
PUBLISHING

Please visit our website, www.garethstevens.com. For a free color catalog of all our high-quality books, call toll free 1-800-542-2595 or fax 1-877-542-2596.

Library of Congress Cataloging-in-Publication Data

Names: Franco, Michou, author.
Title: I'm going to be a doctor! / Michou Franco.
Description: Buffalo, NY : Gareth Stevens Publishing, [2025] | Series: That's the job for me! | Includes index.
Identifiers: LCCN 2023035534 (print) | LCCN 2023035535 (ebook) | ISBN 9781538293294 (library binding) | ISBN 9781538293287 (paperback) | ISBN 9781538293300 (ebook)
Subjects: LCSH: Physicians–Vocational guidance–Juvenile literature.
Classification: LCC R690 .F7137 2025 (print) | LCC R690 (ebook) | DDC 610.69/5–dc23/eng/20230824
LC record available at https://lccn.loc.gov/2023035534
LC ebook record available at https://lccn.loc.gov/2023035535

Published in 2025 by
Gareth Stevens Publishing
2544 Clinton Street
Buffalo, NY 14224

Designer: Claire Zimmermann
Editor: Therese Shea

Photo credits: Cover, pp. 1 Treerat Wongvorapat/Shutterstock.com; Series Art (background) Salmanalfa/Shutterstock.com; pp. 5, 19 fizkes/Shutterstock.com; p. 7 Inside Creative House/Shutterstock.com; p. 9 mrmohock/Shutterstock.com; p. 11 ESB Professional/Shutterstock.com; p. 13 antoniodiaz/Shutterstock.com; p. 15 CandyBox Images/Shutterstock.com; p. 17 I AM NIKOM/Shutterstock.com; p. 21 PIMNADA/Shutterstock.com.

Printed in the United States of America

CPSIA compliance information: Batch #CS25GS: For further information contact Gareth Stevens, New York, New York at 1-800-542-2595.

CONTENTS

Boldface words appear in the glossary.

Becoming a Doctor

I like taking care of people. I like to make them feel better when they're sick or hurt. I'm interested in how people's bodies work. I like to figure out mysteries too. So, I'm going to be a doctor.

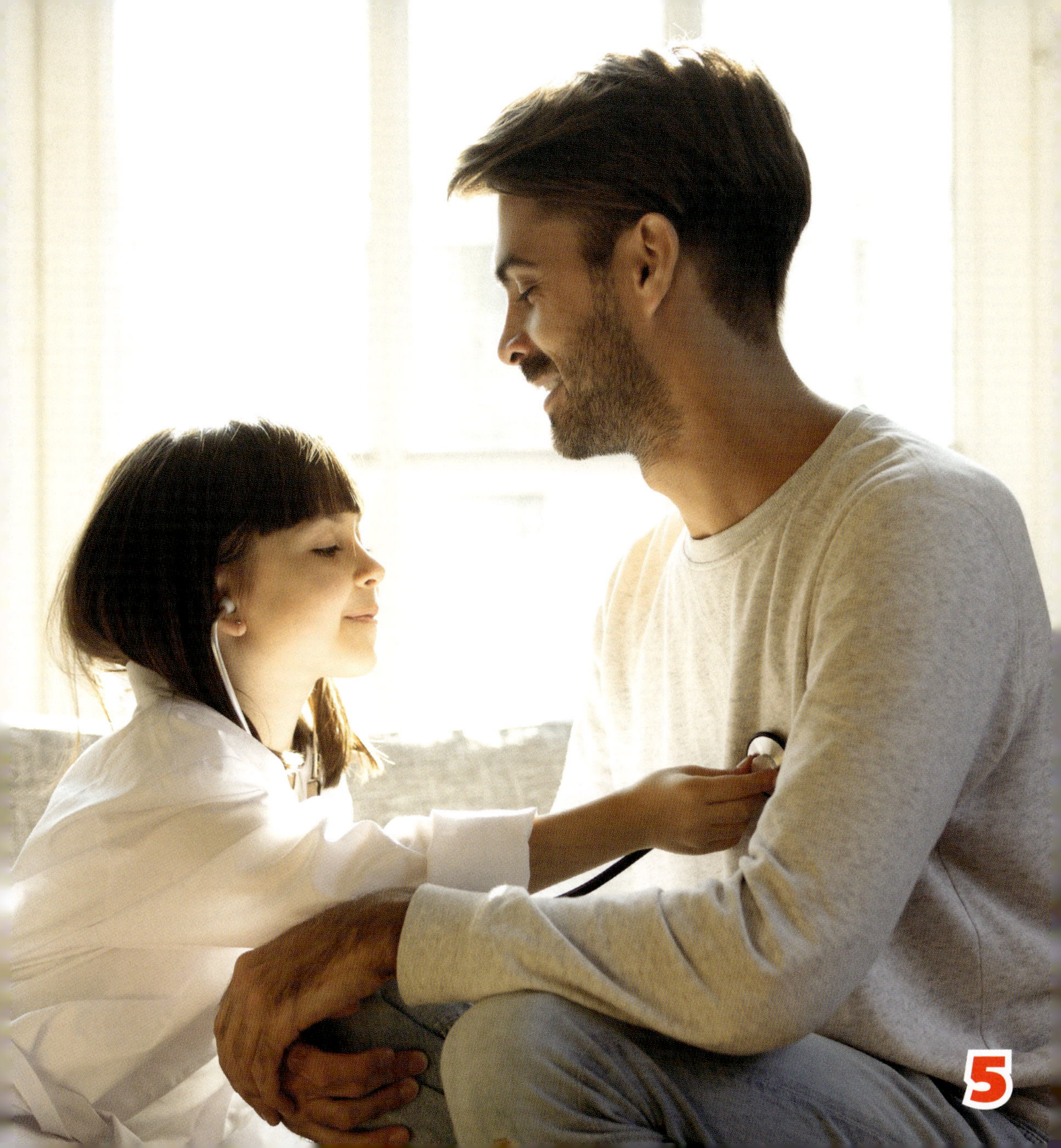

School First

I'll start out by studying in school. Science classes are really important. I'll learn how different body parts work. I'll learn how different body systems work too. The respiratory (REH-spih-reh-tor-ee) system moves air into and out of the **lungs**. Wow!

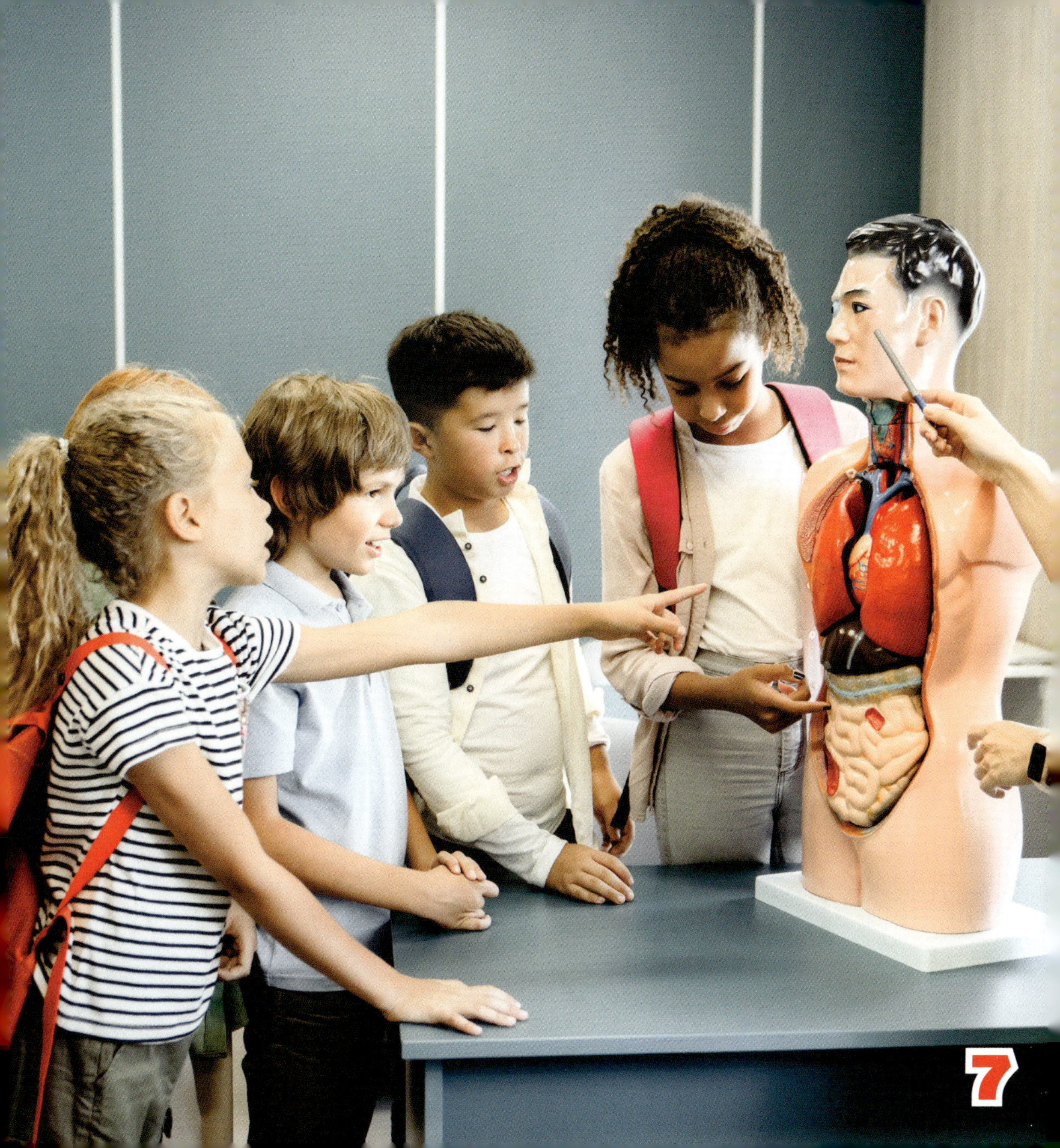

After high school, I'll go to college. I'll take certain classes, such as biology and chemistry. Biology is the study of living things. Chemistry is the study of matter, its **properties**, and how it changes. I'll do **experiments** in a lab!

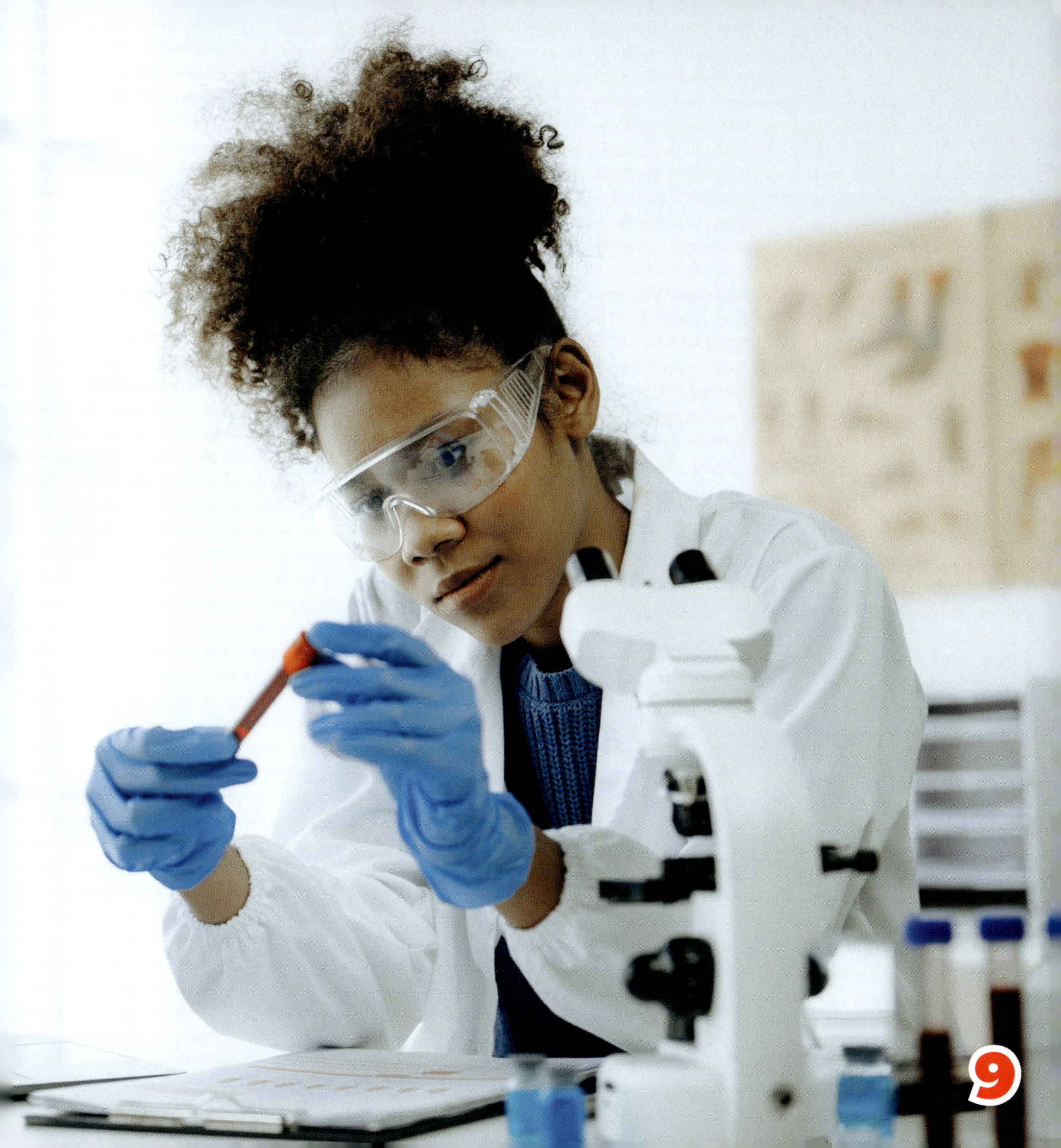

Next is **medical** school. That's another four years. The first two years are in classrooms and labs. The last two years are in **hospitals** and clinics. Medical students work with patients. They learn to do some **procedures** too.

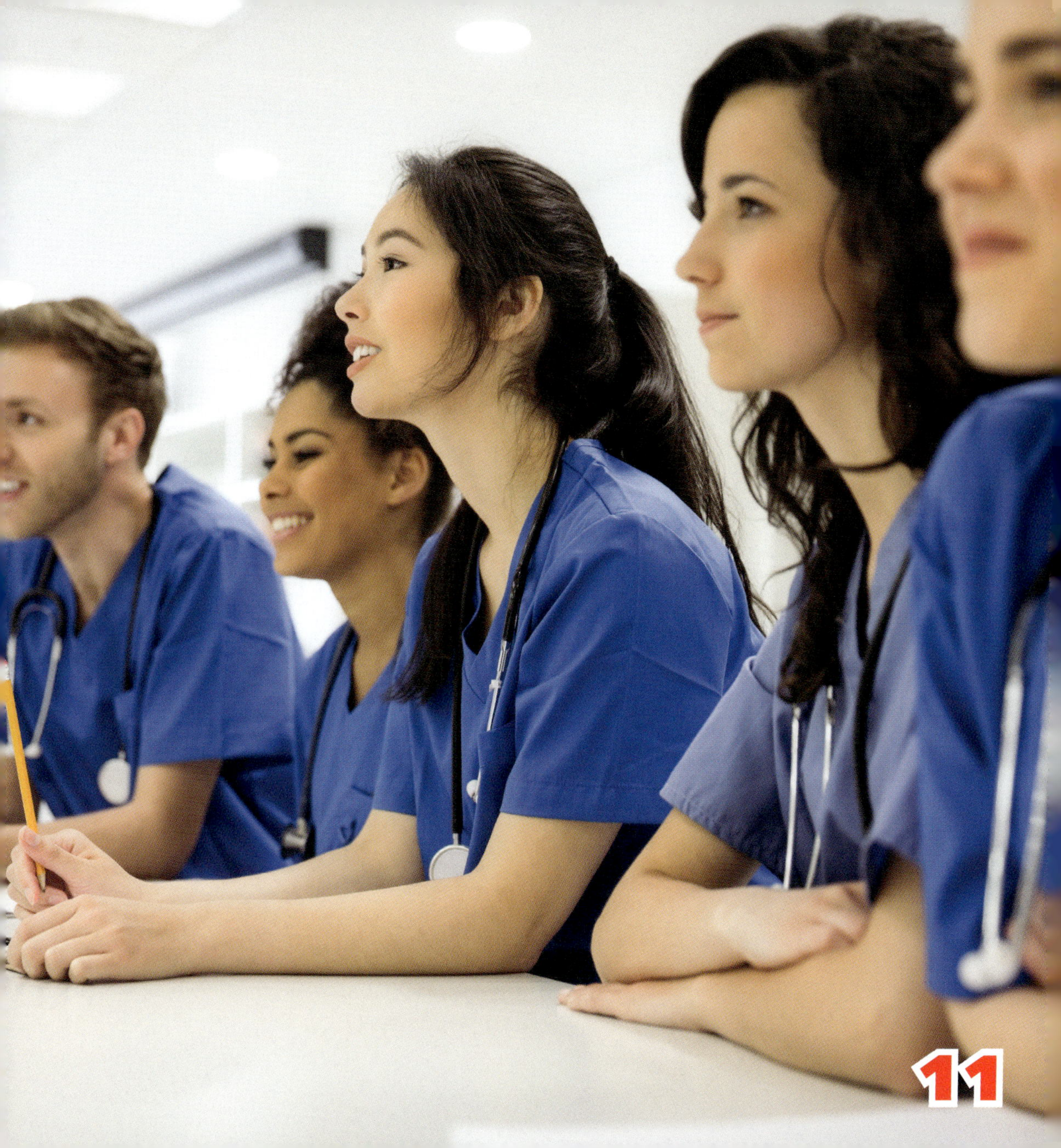

An MD

After medical school, I'll be a doctor of medicine, or an MD. But the studying and learning isn't over. Doctors have a training period called residency for another three to seven years. They **focus** on a medical field.

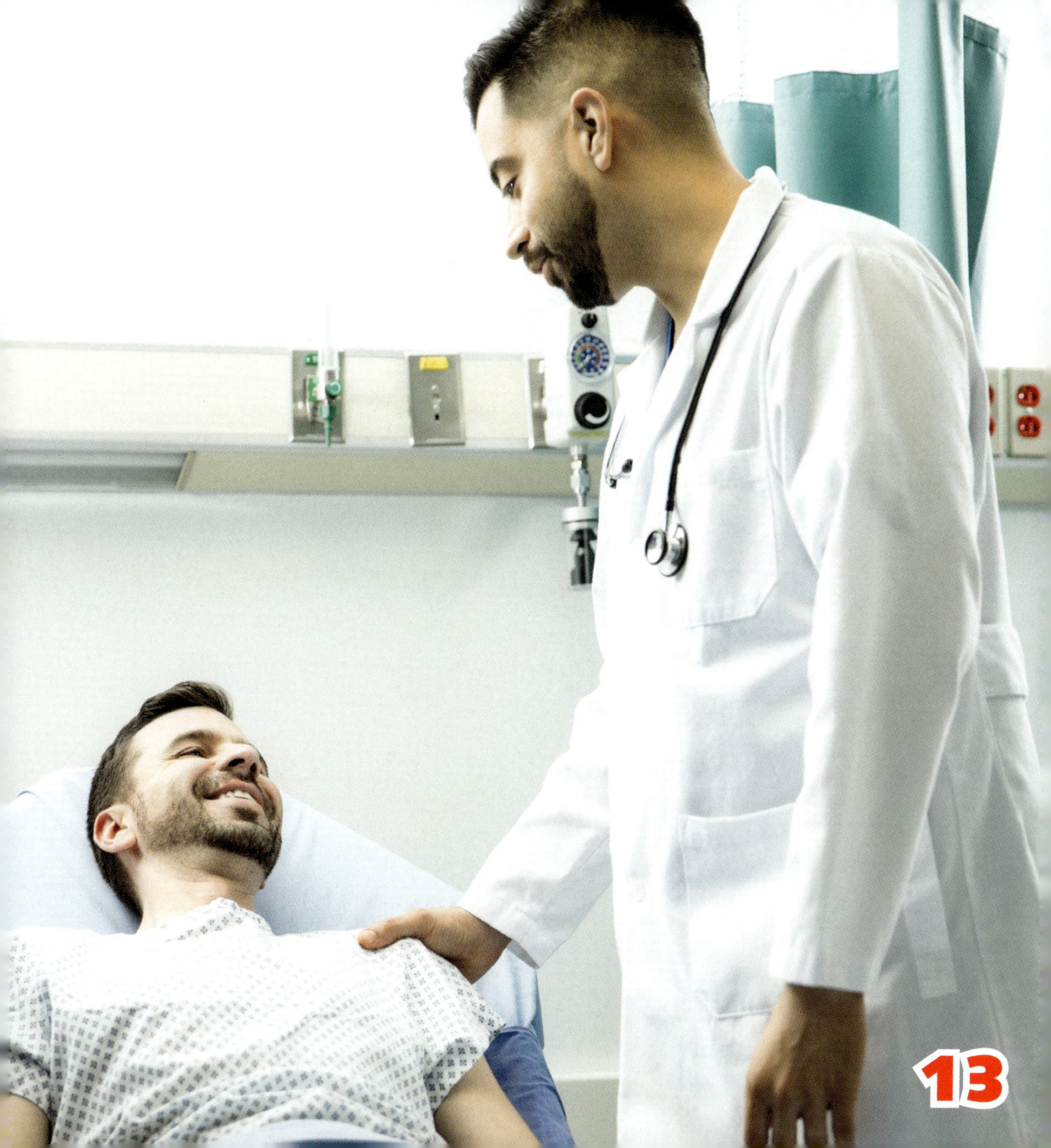

Many Kinds of Doctors

There are hundreds of kinds of doctors! Pediatricians are doctors who take care of babies and children. Cardiologists take care of people's hearts. Surgeons cut into the body to fix body parts. Doctors specialize, or focus on, eyes, skin, bones, and other body parts too.

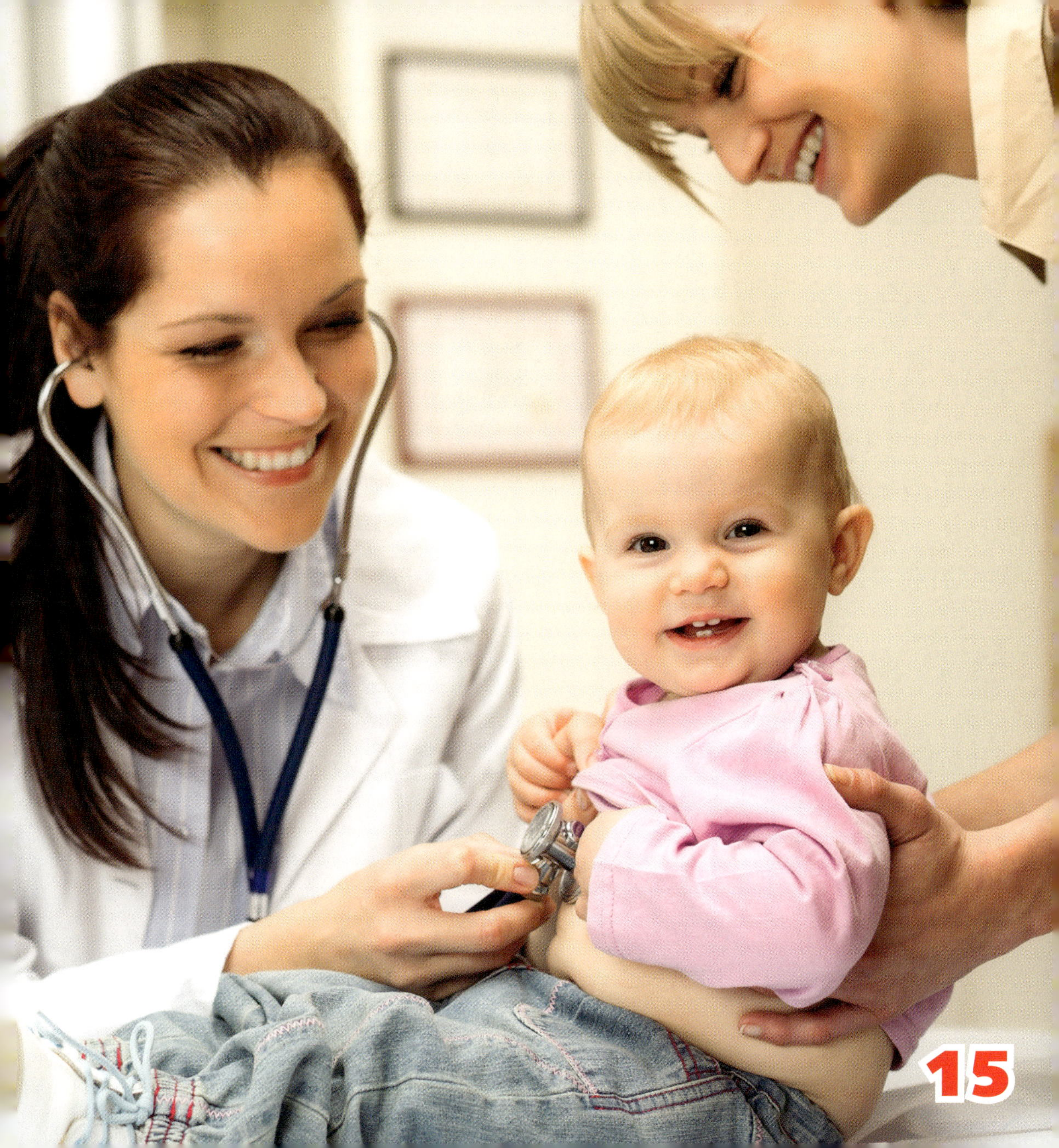

Where Will I Work?

After my residency is done, I'll decide where I want to be a doctor. Will I work in a big hospital? Will I work in a small clinic? I might travel to other countries to help people. I can change jobs too!

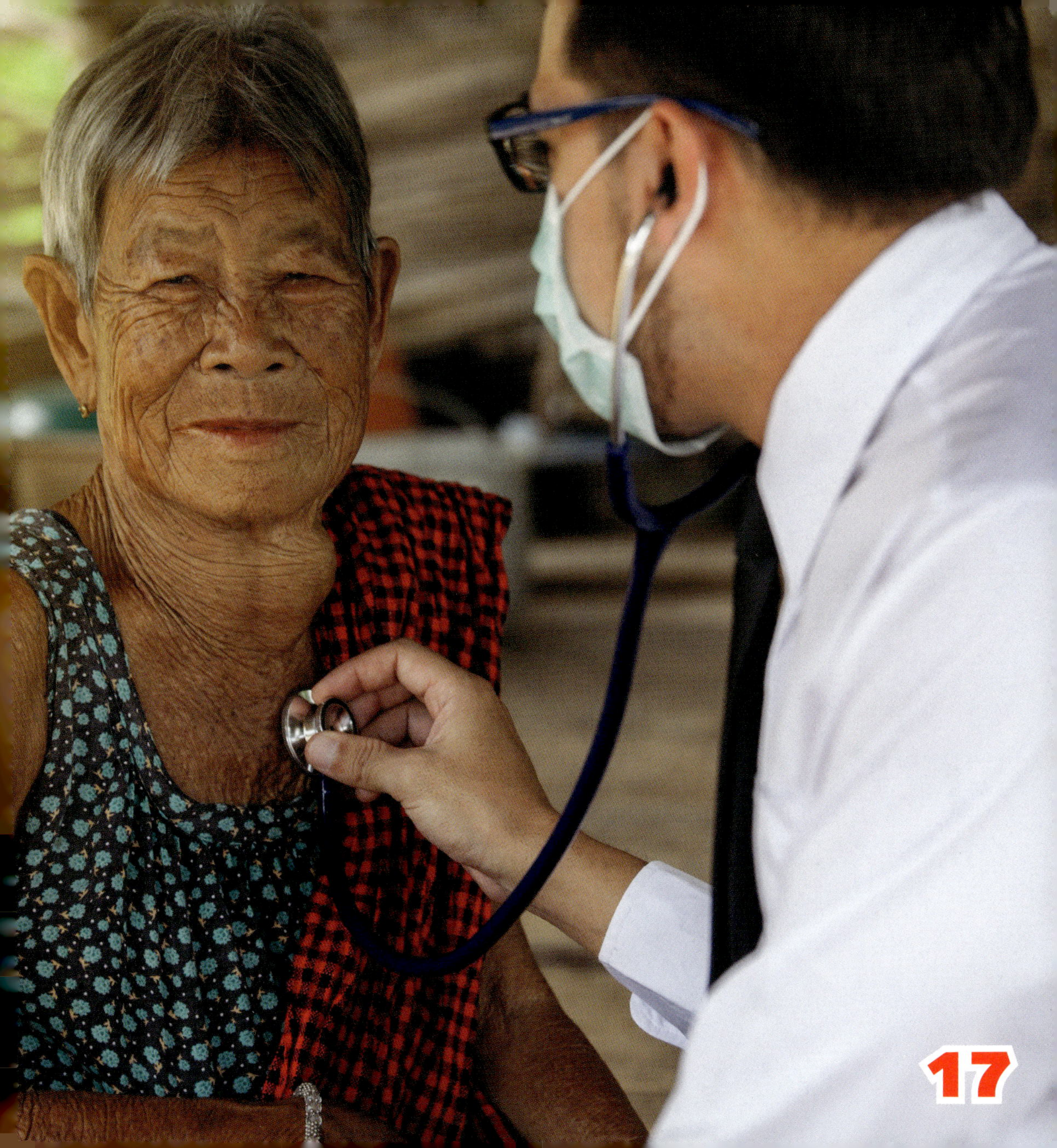

People Skills

A good doctor needs to have certain skills. You can't learn all of these in a classroom. I must be a good listener. I need to listen to what patients tell me. I also need to know what questions to ask.

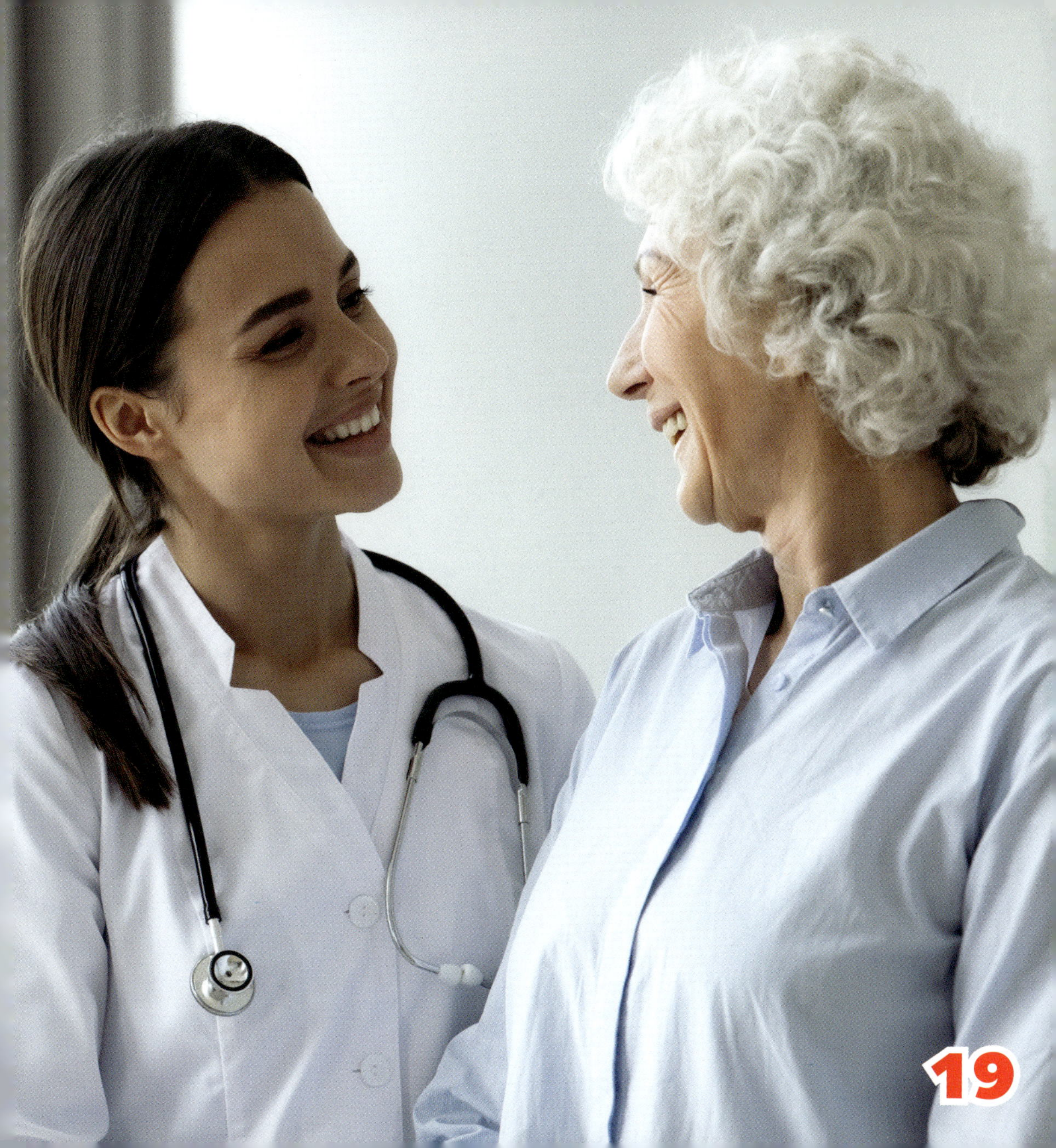

A doctor needs to **communicate** well. They need their patients to understand what they're saying. Doctors also work with nurses and many others. It's important to be a good teammate. I can practice these skills now for the future!

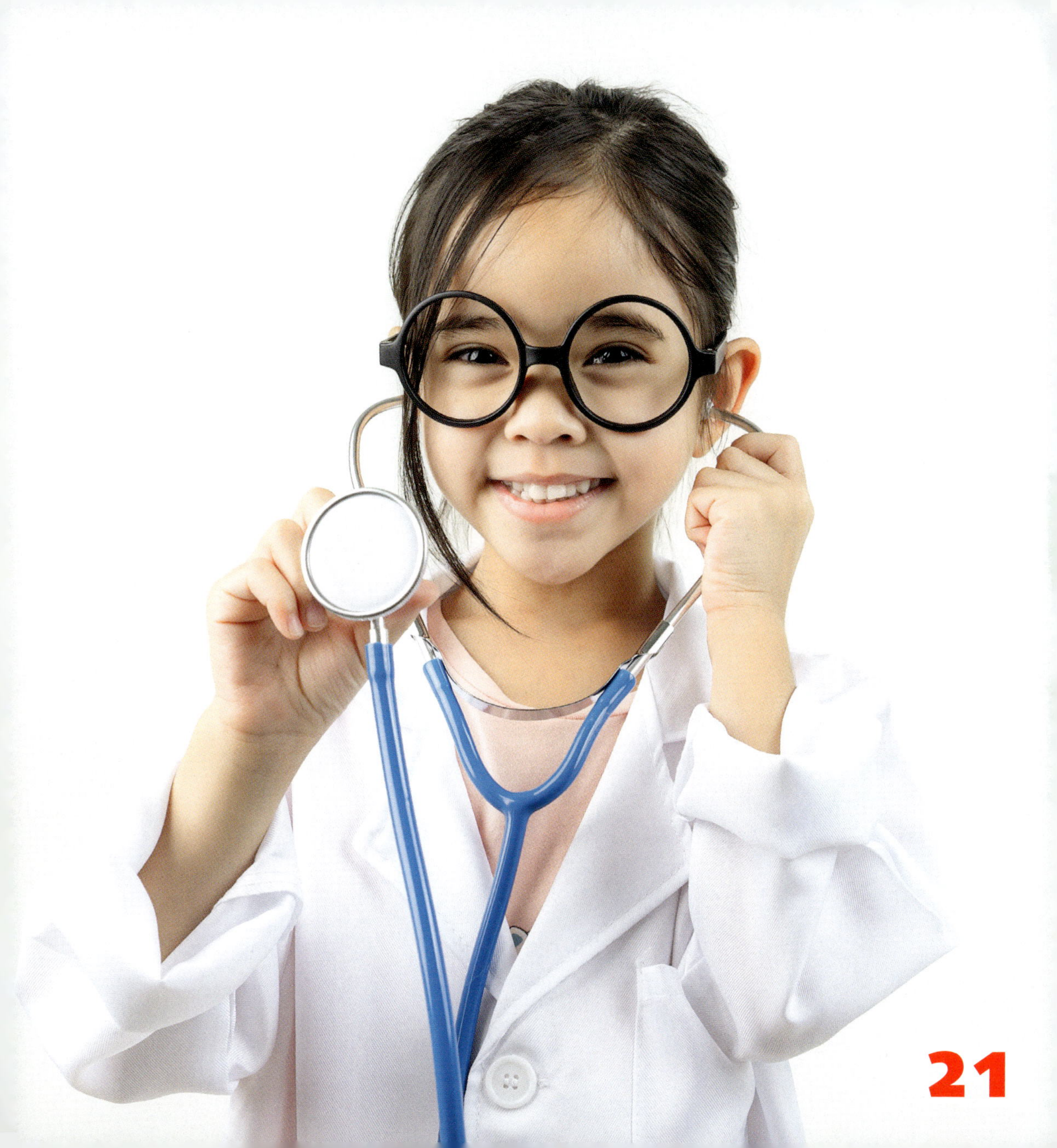

GLOSSARY

communicate: To share ideas and feelings through sounds and motions.

experiment: A scientific test in which you carry out a series of actions and watch what happens in order to learn about something.

focus: To direct your effort to something.

hospital: A place where ill or injured people are given care and where babies are often born.

lung: A part of an animal that takes in air when it breathes.

medical: Having to do with care given by doctors.

procedure: An operation or other medical treatment.

property: A special quality or feature of something.

FOR MORE INFORMATION

BOOKS

Bender, Douglas. *Doctor.* New York, NY: Crabtree Publishing Company, 2022.

Herrick, Becky. *Meet a Doctor!* New York, NY: Children's Press, 2021.

Waxman, Laura Hamilton. *Doctor Tools.* Minneapolis, MN: Lerner Publications, 2020.

WEBSITES

Medical School Facts for Kids
kids.kiddle.co/Medical_school
Doctors go to school for many years! Read about these special schools here.

STEM Career Inspiration: Doctors
blocksrock.com/news-and-learning/stem-career-inspiration-doctors
Read more about different kinds of doctors.

INDEX